CASE STUDIES IN
PUBLIC HEALTH NURSING
ONLINE PRACTICE AND APPLICATION

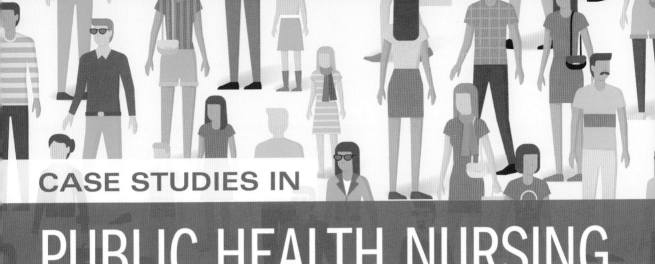

CASE STUDIES IN
PUBLIC HEALTH NURSING
ONLINE PRACTICE AND APPLICATION

Edited by

LISA TURNER, PHD, RN, PHCNS-BC
Associate Professor
Nursing
Berea College
Berea, Kentucky

ELSEVIER

Elsevier
3251 Riverport Lane
St. Louis, Missouri 63043

> **Notice**
>
> Practitioners and researchers must always rely on their own experience and knowledge in evaluating and using any information, methods, compounds or experiments described herein. Because of rapid advances in the medical sciences, in particular, independent verification of diagnoses and drug dosages should be made. To the fullest extent of the law, no responsibility is assumed by Elsevier, authors, editors or contributors for any injury and/or damage to persons or property as a matter of products liability, negligence or otherwise, or from any use or operation of any methods, products, instructions, or ideas contained in the material herein.

International Standard Book Number: 978-0-323-55468-8

Senior Content Strategist: Jamie L. Blum
Senior Content Development Specialist: Tina A. Kaemmerer
Publishing Services Manager: Shereen Jameel
Senior Project Manager: Umarani Natarajan
Design Direction: Brian Salisbury

Printed in China

Last digit is the print number: 9 8 7 6 5 4 3 2 1

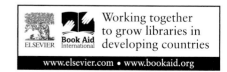

Preface

The scenarios in *Case Studies in Public Health Nursing* are designed to exemplify a broad range of knowledge, skills, and attitudes for promoting population health and practice in community/public health nursing. These unfolding case studies are written for undergraduate nursing students to enhance their comprehension of population health topics, such as community assessment, health promotion, and vulnerable populations, by placing the topic in the context of a public health nursing practice situation. As each case study unfolds, students answer critical thinking questions related to the situation at hand. Each case study incorporates evidence-based practice and exemplifies public health nursing interventions from the Intervention Wheel (Public Health Nursing Section, 2001).

The Quad Council Coalition's [QCC] (2018) *Community/Public Health Nursing [C/PHN] Competencies* was used to provide a framework for the case studies to ensure practice examples for each competency domain were addressed. There are three to six case studies for each domain listed in the *Competencies* document. Pertinent definitions used in the *Competencies* document, such as population health and public health nursing, were also used to guide this work. Case studies that introduce students to working in population health, with select vulnerable populations, and in specialty areas are also included.

Relevant concepts for nursing practice are listed for each case study to help facilitate conceptual learning. The concepts listed match those presented in Giddens, J. (2017). *Concepts for Nursing Practice* (2nd ed.). St. Louis: Elsevier.

Each case study provides suggested readings from textbooks related to population health and public/community health nursing. The case studies can be used alone or in conjunction with these texts.

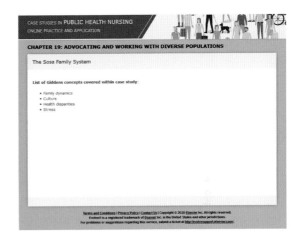

Each case study begins with a synopsis and a list of objectives. The objectives identify the primary goals of learning for the case study.

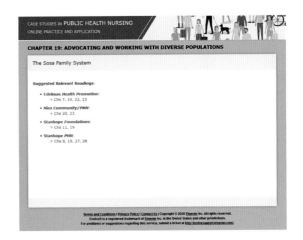

An estimated completion time is provided for each case study. Use this as a guide when preparing to work through the case study. Be sure to allow yourself enough time to read through the case study and answer any related questions.

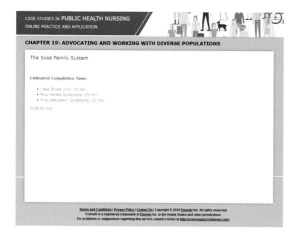

NOTE FOR INSTRUCTORS

Critical thinking questions are interspersed throughout the case study. Answers for multiple choice and multiple response questions will be recorded in the gradebook, and immediate feedback with rationales will be provided for students. Immediate feedback will also be provided for short-answer questions, but grading is not automatic. A "Review Mode" section at the end provides the option to print or save results so students can submit detailed summaries of their work.

An Instructor Facilitator Guide is available online to provide additional guidance for utilizing the case studies in your curriculum.

REFERENCES

Giddens, J. (2017). *Concepts for Nursing Practice* (ed. 2). St. Louis, MO: Elsevier.

Quad Council Coalition Competency Review Task Force. (2018). *Community/Public Health Nursing Competencies*. Retrieved from http://www.quadcouncilphn.org/documents-3/2018-qcc-competencies/.

Section, Public Health Nursing. (2001). *Public Health Interventions: Applications for Public Health Nursing Practice*. St. Paul: Minnesota Dept. of Health. Retrieved from http://www.health.state.mn.us/divs/opi/cd/phn/wheel. html.

Contributors

Karen Alexander, PhD, BSN, AAS
Director, Assistant Professor RN-BSN
Nursing
University of Houston Clear Lake
Houston, Texas

Karen Britt, DNP
Assistant Professor
Nursing
MCPHS University
Manchester, New Hampshire

Maryanne Capp, DNP, RN
Chair
Nursing
Wheeling Jesuit University
Wheeling, West Virginia

Lois A. Davis, MSN, MA
Public Health Clinical Instructor
College of Nursing
University of Kentucky
Lexington, Kentucky

Janice Ann Edelstein, EdD, MSN, MEd, BSN
Associate Professor
Nursing Department
Marian University
Fond du Lac, Wisconsin
Nursing Instructor
Nursing
Wisconsin Lutheran College
Milwaukee, Wisconsin

Sharon Farra, PhD, RN
Associate Professor
Nursing
Wright State University
Dayton, Ohio

Hartley Carmichael Feld, PhD, MSN
Nursing Faculty
College of Nursing
University of Kentucky
Lexington, Kentucky

Monty Gross, PhD, MSN, BSN, BS
Senior Nurse Leader for Professional Development
Nursing Administration
Health Services Authority
George Town, Cayman Islands

Karen Ivantic, DNP, RN, FNP-BC
Professor
Nursing
Columbia College of Nursing
Glendale, Wisconsin
Owner/Director
NP Consults LLC
Milwaukee, Wisconsin

Lisa Jaurigue, PhD, MSN-Ed, BSN
Clinical Assistant Professor
College of Nursing and Health Innovation
Arizona State University
Phoenix, Arizona
Fellow
Integrative Nursing Faculty Fellowship
University of Arizona
Tucson, Arizona

Ericka Kalp, PhD, MPH, CIC, FAPIC
Director
Epidemiology and Infection Prevention
Summit Health
Chambersburg, Pennsylvania

Loren S. Kelly, MSN, BA,ADN
Clinician Educator/Faculty
Nursing
UNM College of Nursing, Albuquerque
Albuquerque, New Mexico

Dawn Koonkongsatian, MSN-Ed, RN
Lecturer
School of Nursing
Nevada State College
Henderson, Nevada

Connie Lamb, PhD, MSN, BSN
Associate Professor
Nursing
Berea College
Berea, Kentucky

Susan K. Lee, PhD, MSN, BSN
Nursing Consultant for Education
Nursing
Austin, Texas

Gail McGillis, MSN
Chief Executive Officer
Administration
Hospice Care Plus
Berea, Kentucky

Carol McLay, DrPH, MPH, RN, CIC, FAPIC
CEO
Infection Control International
Chapel Hill, North Carolina

Judy Ponder, DNP, RN-BC
Director of Education and Professional Development
Education and Professional Development
Baptist Health Richmond
Richmond, Kentucky

Sherrill Smith, PhD, MS, BSN
Assistant Dean for Undergraduate Programs
College of Nursing and Health
Wright State University
Dayton, Ohio

Marcia Stanhope, PhD, RN, FAAN
Professor Emeritus
College of Nursing
University of Kentucky
Lexington, Kentucky

Leigh Ann Tovar, MSN-Ed, MAOM, RN-BC, CNE
Adjunct Professor
Nursing
Arizona State University
Grand Canyon University
Phoenix, Arizona

Lisa Turner, PhD, RN, PHCNS-BC
Associate Professor
Nursing
Berea College
Berea, Kentucky

Christine Varner, MSN, CSN
Nursing Instructor
Health Sciences
Mansfield University
Mansfield, Pennsylvania
Staff Nurse
Emergency Department
Guthrie Towanda Memorial Hospital
Towanda, Pennsylvania

Margie Washnok, BAN, MS, DNP
Nursing
Presentation College
Aberdeen, South Dakota

Pamela Willson, PhD, APRN, FNP-BC, CNE, FAANP
Director of Graduate Education
School of Nursing
Texas State University
Round Rock, Texas

Susan E. Young, PhD, BSN
Assistant Professor
School of Nursing
Florida Gulf Coast University
Fort Myers, Florida

Janet Zoellner, BSN, MS
Nursing Instructor
Health Sciences
Blackhawk Technical College
Janesville, Wisconsin

Contents

CASE STUDY 1

Upstream Thinking
Introduction to Public Health Nursing

Case Study Synopsis: Nurse Jamie is an emergency department nurse investigating the sudden increase in teenage driver motor vehicle accidents.

Estimated Completion Time:
- Case study only: 1 hour
- Plus review questions: + 30 minutes
- Plus discussion questions: + 30 minutes
- Total: 2 hours

Concepts Covered:
- Leadership
- Health promotion
- Health policy

Public Health Nursing Interventions Addressed:
- Surveillance
- Health teaching
- Advocacy
- Policy development and enforcement

Suggested Readings:
- **Edelman and Kudzma's** *Health Promotion Throughout the Life Span*
  - Chapter 1: Health Defined: Objectives for Promotion and Prevention
  - Chapter 21: Adolescent

- **Nies and McEwen's** *Community/Public Health Nursing*
  - Chapter 1: Health: A Community View
  - Chapter 3: Thinking Upstream: Nursing Theories and Population-Focused Nursing Practice
- **Stanhope and Lancaster's** *Foundations for Population Health in Community/Public Health Nursing*
  - Chapter 1: Community- and Prevention-Oriented Practice to Improve Population Health
- **Stanhope and Lancaster's** *Public Health Nursing*
  - Chapter 1: Public Health Foundations and Population Health

Case Study Objectives:
After completing this case study, the student should be able to:
1. Differentiate upstream and downstream interventions.
2. Differentiate community health nursing, public health nursing, community-oriented nursing, and community-based nursing.
3. Analyze data in assessing a problem in the community.
4. Apply the nursing process at the community level.

Determinants of Health

Case Study Synopsis: A public health nurse is working on a grant application focusing on obesity and needs to identify the determinants of health in community that influence this issue.

Estimated Completion Time:
- Case study only: 1 hour
- Plus review questions: + 30 minutes
- Plus discussion questions: + 30 minutes
- Total: 2 hours

Concepts Covered:
- Leadership
- Health promotion
- Health policy

Public Health Nursing Interventions Addressed:
- Advocacy
- Surveillance
- Screening health teaching
- Disease and other health event investigations
- Coalition building
- Policy development

Suggested Readings:
- **Edelman and Kudzma's** *Health Promotion Throughout the Life Span*
  - Chapter 1: Health Defined: Objectives for Promotion and Prevention
- **Nies and McEwen's** *Community/Public Health Nursing*
  - Chapter 1: Health: A Community View
  - Chapter 3: Thinking Upstream: Nursing Theories and Population-Focused Nursing Practice
- **Stanhope and Lancaster's** *Foundations for Population Health in Community/Public Health Nursing*
  - Chapter 1: Community- and Prevention-Oriented Practice to Improve Population Health
  - Chapter 21: Vulnerability and Vulnerable Populations: An Overview
- **Stanhope and Lancaster's** *Public Health Nursing*
  - Chapter 1: Public Health Foundations and Population Health
  - Chapter 16: Promoting Healthy Communities
  - Chapter 17: Community as Client: Assessment and Analysis
  - Chapter 31: Vulnerability and Vulnerable Populations: An Overview

Case Study Objectives:
After completing this case study, the student should be able to:
1. Describe population groups who might be considered vulnerable.
2. Identify the ways vulnerable populations often have health disparities compared with the general population.
3. Examine individual and social factors that may contribute to vulnerability.

Culture of Health

Case Study Synopsis: A public health nurse leads an interdisciplinary team that is challenged to initially improve the health of their service delivery area after seeing a rise in chronic diseases such as diabetes and heart disease. However, the team soon realizes that they need to think more broadly about health. The case unfolds using the public health core functions, the public health nursing intervention wheel, and the Robert Wood Johnson Foundation's call to action to change the culture of health.

Estimated Completion Time:
- Case study only: 2 hours
- Plus review questions: + 30 minutes
- Plus discussion questions: + 30 minutes
- Total: 3 hours

Concepts Covered:
- Health policy
- Health disparities
- Collaboration
- Clinical judgment
- Leadership
- Ethics
- Health promotion
- Culture
- Stress

Public Health Nursing Interventions Addressed:
- Surveillance
- Collaboration
- Community organization building
- Advocacy
- Policy development

Suggested Readings:
- **Nies and McEwen's** *Community/Public Health Nursing*
  - Chapter 1: Health: A Community View
  - Chapter 3: Thinking Upstream: Nursing Theories and Population-Focused Nursing Practice
  - Chapter 6: Community Assessment
  - Chapter 10: Policy, Politics, Legislations, and Community Health Nursing
  - Chapter 13: Cultural Diversity and Community Health Nursing
  - Chapter 14: Environmental Health
- **Stanhope and Lancaster's** *Foundations for Population Health in Community/Public Health Nursing*
  - Chapter 1: Community- and Prevention-Oriented Practice to Improved Population Health
- **Stanhope and Lancaster's** *Public Health Nursing*
  - Chapter 1: Public Health Foundations and Population Health
  - Chapter 11: Population-Based Public Health Nursing Practice: The Intervention Wheel
  - Chapter 18: Building a Culture of Health to Influence Health Equity within Communities

Case Study Objectives:
After completing this case study, the student should be able to:
1. Apply theoretical and action frameworks to broaden our understanding of health.
2. Identify how the culture of health framework integrates with the public health core competencies and the PHN wheel.
3. Identify the components of the intervention wheel to create an action plan.
4. Envision a broader role of nurse leadership, advocacy, and collaboration with non-health sectors in the community.

CASE STUDY 4

Community Assessment Part 1
Shoe Leather/Windshield Survey and Key Informant Interview

Case Study Synopsis: As a public health nurse, you have been contacted and asked to conduct a community assessment as part of an updated strategic plan for future growth and development in a nearby community. You know that this is an opportunity to find the strengths and weaknesses of the community, and to offer suggestions for improvement of the overall health and wellness of the population.

Estimated Completion Time:
- Case study only: 2 hours
- Plus review questions: + 30 minutes
- Plus discussion questions: + 1 hour
- Total: 3.5 hours

Concepts Covered:
- Health promotion
- Health policy

Public Health Nursing Interventions Addressed:
- Disease and health event investigation
- Consultation
- Policy development and enforcement

Suggested Readings:
- **Edelman and Kudzma's** *Health Promotion Throughout the Life Span*
  - Chapter 8: Health Promotion and the Community

- **Nies and McEwen's** *Community/Public Health Nursing*
  - Chapter 6: Community Assessment
- **Stanhope and Lancaster's** *Foundations for Population Health in Community/Public Health Nursing*
  - Chapter 12: Community Assessment and Evaluation
- **Stanhope and Lancaster's** *Public Health Nursing*
  - Chapter 17: Community as Client: Assessment and Analysis

Case Study Objectives:
After completing this case study, the student should be able to:
1. Identify relevant and appropriate data and information sources to better understand the community being assessed.
2. Gather demographic, geographic, governmental, health care, cultural, and socioeconomic data of the community.
3. Conduct a preliminary analysis of data collected in the windshield survey and community assessment to identify strengths and weaknesses of the community.
4. Propose recommendations for a strategic plan based on the results of the community assessment.

Community Assessment Part 2
Using Data Sources

Case Study Synopsis: A public health nurse conducted a community assessment, collecting data and interviewing stakeholders, and completing a windshield survey (see Case Study 4). In this case study, the collected data will be analyzed for presenting findings to the stakeholders and a final written report will include risk factors, issues, and suggestions for potential solutions.

Estimated Completion Time:
- Case study only: 2 hours
- Plus review questions: + 45 minutes
- Plus discussion questions: + 45 minutes
- Total: 3.5 hours

Concepts Covered:
- Professionalism
- Clinical judgment
- Health promotion
- Evidence
- Health care quality
- Care coordination
- Health care economics
- Health policy

Public Health Nursing Interventions Addressed:
- Surveillance
- Disease and other health event investigation
- Outreach
- Health teaching
- Consultation
- Collaboration
- Coalition building
- Community organizing
- Policy development and enforcement

Suggested Readings:
- Edelman and Kudzma's *Health Promotion Throughout the Life Span*
  - Chapter 8: Health Promotion and the Community
  - Chapter 10: Health Education
- Nies and McEwen's *Community/Public Health Nursing*
  - Chapter 6: Community Assessment
  - Chapter 7: Community Health Planning, Implementation, and Evaluation
  - Chapter 14: Environmental Health
- Stanhope and Lancaster's *Foundations for Population Health in Community/Public Health Nursing*
  - Chapter 1: Community- and Prevention-Oriented Practice to Improve Population Health
  - Chapter 10: Evidence-Based Practice
  - Chapter 11: Using Health Education and Groups in the Community
  - Chapter 12: Community Assessment and Evaluation
- Stanhope and Lancaster's *Public Health Nursing*
  - Chapter 6: Environmental Health
  - Chapter 10: Evidence-Based Practice
  - Chapter 11: Population-Based Public Health Nursing Practice: The Intervention Wheel
  - Chapter 17: Community as Client: Assessment and Analysis

Case Study Objectives:
After completing this case study, the student should be able to:
1. Describe the role of public health nursing in population and community health.
2. Discuss how the role of the public health nurse influences the community.
3. Analyze the impact of evidence-based practice on the community.
4. Identify the 11 functional health patterns that are used during data collection in community assessments.
5. Discuss potential dysfunctional health patterns.
6. Describe methods of planned change for communities.
7. Make recommendations for community improvement using evidence-based practice.
8. Identify barriers to evidence-based practice in the community.
9. Identify methods in which public health nurses can work with community members and stakeholders to promote community health.
10. Apply methods of assessment, recommend interventions, and evaluate community situations to promote community health.
11. Develop a health-promotion plan based on the community assessment conducted in Case Study 4.

Individual Health Risk Assessment

Case Study Synopsis: This case study illustrates that health risk assessments can be complex when considering family genetics and multiple disease conditions.

Estimated Completion Time:
- Case study only: 15 minutes
- Plus review questions: + 20 minutes
- Plus discussion questions: + 20 minutes
- Total: 55 minutes

Concepts Covered:
- Self-management
- Patient education
- Glucose regulation
- Perfusion

Public Health Nursing Interventions Addressed:
- Screening
- Referral and follow-up
- Health teaching
- Counseling

Suggested Readings:
- **Edelman and Kudzma's** *Health Promotion Throughout the Life Span*
  - Chapter 6: Health Promotion and the Individual
  - Chapter 10: Health Education
- **Nies and McEwen's** *Community/Public Health Nursing*
  - Chapter 4: Health Promotion and Risk Reduction
  - Chapter 8: Community Health Education
  - Chapter 30: School Health
- **Stanhope and Lancaster's** *Foundations for Population Health in Community/Public Health Nursing*
  - Chapter 20: Health Risks Across the Lifespan
  - Chapter 21: Vulnerability and Vulnerable Populations: An Overview
- **Stanhope and Lancaster's** *Public Health Nursing*
  - Chapter 29: Major Health Issues and Chronic Disease Management of Adults Across the Life Span
  - Chapter 31: Vulnerability and Vulnerable Populations

Case Study Objectives:

After completing this case study, the student should be able to:

1. Describe considerations and strategies leading to a successful health risk assessment for an individual.
2. Complete a comprehensive health risk assessment on an individual.
3. Identify major risks for individuals.
4. Describe screening tools appropriate for various age groups.
5. Describe major components in an individual health risk assessment tool(s).

Family Health Risk Assessment

Case Study Synopsis: This case study illustrates the family health risks of the Sosa family and influences of systems on health.

Estimated Completion Time:
- Case study only: 15 minutes
- Plus review questions: + 25 minutes
- Plus discussion questions: + 20 minutes
- Total: 60 minutes

Concepts Covered:
- Family dynamics
- Culture
- Health disparities
- Stress

Public Health Nursing Interventions Addressed:
- Community organization
- Consultation
- Health teaching
- Referral and follow-up

Suggested Readings:
- **Edelman and Kudzma's** *Health Promotion Throughout the Life Span*
  - Chapter 7: Health Promotion and the Individual
  - Chapter 10: Health Education
  - Chapter 22: Young Adult
  - Chapter 23: Middle-Age Adult
- **Nies and McEwen's** *Community/Public Health Nursing*
  - Chapter 20: Family Health
  - Chapter 24: Rural and Migrant Health
- **Stanhope and Lancaster's** *Foundations for Population Health in Community/Public Health Nursing*
  - Chapter 11: Using Health Education and Groups in the Community
  - Chapter 19: Family Health Risks
- **Stanhope and Lancaster's** *Public Health Nursing*
  - Chapter 9: Public Health Policy
  - Chapter 26: Working with Families in the Community for Healthy Outcomes
  - Chapter 27: Family Health Risks

Case Study Objectives:
After completing this case study, the student should be able to:
1. Perform a health risk assessment for a family.
2. Relate a systems theory perspective to the case information provided.
3. Complete a genogram and an ecomap using the information provided.

Environmental Health Risk Assessment

Case Study Synopsis: This case study illustrates environmental health risks and the role of community health nurses. It also explores the impact of war, immigration, and health disparities.

Estimated Completion Time:
- Case study only: 15 minutes
- Plus review questions: + 25 minutes
- Plus discussion questions: + 20 minutes
- Total: 1 hour

Concepts Covered:
- Culture
- Health disparities
- Safety
- Stress

Public Health Nursing Interventions Addressed:
- Advocacy
- Community organization
- Coalition building
- Policy development and enforcement

Suggested Readings:
- Edelman and Kudzma's *Health Promotion Throughout the Life Span*
  - Chapter 7: Health Promotion and the Individual
- Nies and McEwen's *Community/Public Health Nursing*
  - Chapter 6: Community Assessment
  - Chapter 14: Environmental Health
- Stanhope and Lancaster's *Foundations for Population Health in Community/Public Health Nursing*
  - Chapter 6: Environmental Health
  - Chapter 20: Health Risks Across the Life Span
- Stanhope and Lancaster's *Public Health Nursing*
  - Chapter 6: Environmental Health
  - Chapter 7: Application of Ethics in the Community

Case Study Objectives:

After completing this case study, the student should be able to:

1. Explore aspects of social or environmental justice in relation to communities.
2. Describe aspects of environmental health.
3. Discuss ways to assess environmental health risk in the community.
4. Recognize social stigma as a factor in community health.

CASE STUDY 9

Policy Development to Protect Health
Local Community Level Policy

Case Study Synopsis: Nurse Amanda is a school nurse working on implementation of a local health policy to prohibit smoking and vaping in outdoor public places.

Estimated Completion Time:
- Case study only: 45 minutes
- Plus review questions: + 15 minutes
- Plus discussion questions: + 30 minutes
- Total: 1.5 hours

Concepts Covered:
- Health policy
- Health care law

List of Public Health Interventions Addressed in Case Study:
- Advocacy
- Heath teaching
- Policy development and enforcement
- Coalition building

Suggested Readings:
- **Edelman and Kudzma's** *Health Promotion Throughout the Life Span*
  - Chapter 3: Health Policy and the Delivery System
- **Nies and McEwen's** *Community/Public Health Nursing*
  - Chapter 10: Policy, Politics, Legislation, and Community Health Nursing
- **Stanhope and Lancaster's** *Foundations for Population Health in Community/Public Health Nursing*
  - Chapter 7: Government, the Law, and Policy Activism
- **Stanhope and Lancaster's** *Public Health Nursing*
  - Chapter 9: Public Health Policy

Case Study Objectives:
After completing this case study, the student should be able to:
1. Understand the process of policy development.
2. Differentiate between cognitive, affective, and psychomotor learning domains.
3. Identify reliable sources of education and data.
4. Recognize the role of coalitions in policy development.
5. Identify levels of prevention in community program planning.
6. Understand advocacy as it relates to policy development.

Policy Development to Protect Health
State Level Policy

Case Study Synopsis: Mary, a nurse case manager in an outpatient clinic, advocates for resources for vulnerable patients.

Estimated Completion Time:
- Case study only: 30 minutes
- Plus review questions: + 15 minutes
- Plus discussion questions: + 15 minutes
- Total: 1 hour

Concepts Covered:
- Leadership
- Communication
- Collaboration
- Care coordination
- Health policy

Public Health Nursing Interventions Addressed:
- Advocacy
- Case management
- Coalition building
- Collaboration
- Policy development and enforcement

Suggested Readings:
- Edelman and Kudzma's *Health Promotion Throughout the Life Span*
  - Chapter 3: Health Policy and the Delivery System
  - Chapter 8: Health Promotion and the Community
- Nies and McEwen's *Community/Public Health Nursing*
  - Chapter 9: Case Management
  - Chapter 10: Policy, Politics, Legislation, and Community Health Nursing
- Stanhope and Lancaster's *Foundations for Population Health in Community/Public Health Nursing*
  - Chapter 7: Government, the Law, and Policy Activism
  - Chapter 13: Case Management
- Stanhope and Lancaster's *Public Health Nursing*
  - Chapter 9: Public Health Policy
  - Chapter 25: Case Management

Case Study Objectives:
After completing this case study, the student should be able to:
1. Identify policy issues and implications relevant to health.
2. Differentiate between legislative and budgeting processes.
3. Discuss strategies for advocating to protect and promote health.
4. Apply the nursing process to health care policy.

Policy Development to Protect Health
National Level Policy

Case Study Synopsis: Josh is a public health nurse advocating for health care services for older members of his small rural community.

Estimated Completion Time:

- Case study only: 30 minutes
- Plus review questions: + 15 minutes
- Plus discussion questions: + 15 minutes
- Total: 1 hour

Concepts Covered:

- Leadership
- Communication
- Collaboration
- Health policy

Public Health Nursing Interventions Addressed:

- Advocacy
- Coalition building
- Collaboration
- Policy development and enforcement

Suggested Readings:

- **Edelman and Kudzma's** *Health Promotion Throughout the Life Span*
  - Chapter 3: Health Policy and the Delivery System
- Chapter 8: Health Promotion and the Community
- **Nies and McEwen's** *Community/Public Health Nursing*
  - Chapter 10: Policy, Politics, Legislation, and Community Health Nursing
- **Stanhope and Lancaster's** *Foundations for Population Health in Community/Public Health Nursing*
  - Chapter 7: Government, the Law, and Policy Activism
- **Stanhope and Lancaster's** *Public Health Nursing*
  - Chapter 9: Public Health Policy

Case Study Objectives:

After completing this case study, the student should be able to:

1. Identify policy issues and implications relevant to the health of communities.
2. Describe the legislative process of how a bill becomes a law.
3. Discuss the nurse's role in advocating for policies that protect and promote health at the national level.
4. Apply the nursing process to health care policy development.

Program Planning

Case Study Synopsis: Margaret, a registered nurse (RN), works in a primary care clinic in a rural community that provides care for families and adults, with a focus on older adults (over age 65) diagnosed with diabetes type 2. Margaret has noticed that an increasing number of patients have poorly controlled diabetes, with HbA1c levels greater than 9, and many express feeling overwhelmed with managing their diabetes effectively at home.

Estimated Completion Time:
- Case study only: 1 hour
- Plus review questions: + 30 minutes
- Plus discussion questions: + 30 minutes
- Total: 2 hours

Concepts Covered:
- Self-management
- Leadership
- Health promotion

Public Health Nursing Interventions Addressed:
- Health teaching
- Referral and follow-up
- Case management
- Advocacy
- Outreach

Suggested Readings:
- **Edelman and Kudzma's** *Health Promotion Throughout the Life Span*
  - Chapter 8: Health Promotion and the Community
- **Nies and McEwen's** *Community/Public Health Nursing*
  - Chapter 7: Community Health Planning, Implementation, and Evaluation
- **Stanhope and Lancaster's** *Foundations for Population Health in Community/Public Health Nursing*
  - Chapter 16: Program Management
- **Stanhope and Lancaster's** *Public Health Nursing*
  - Chapter 23: Program Management

Case Study Objectives:
After completing this case study, the student should be able to:
1. Analyze need for a community health promotion program.
2. Explain the program planning process.
3. Create program goals and objectives.
4. Identify tools for program planning/intervention (i.e., Gantt chart).
5. Plan for evaluation of program.

Disaster Planning and Management Part 1

Mitigation and Preparation

Case Study Synopsis: Nurse Christine Snyder is a home health nurse assisting with the development of a disaster preparation plan as part of her care of an elderly community member.

Estimated Completion Time:
- Case study only: 30 minutes
- Plus review questions: + 20 minutes
- Plus discussion questions: + 10 minutes
- Total: 1 hour

Concepts Covered:
- Patient education
- Safety
- Care coordination

Public Health Nursing Interventions Addressed:
- Advocacy
- Health teaching

Suggested Readings:
- **Edelman and Kudzma's** *Health Promotion Throughout the Life Span*
  - Chapter 25: Health Promotion for the Twenty-First Century: Throughout the Lifespan and Throughout the World
- **Nies and McEwen's** *Community/Public Health Nursing*
  - Chapter 29: Natural and Man-Made Disasters
- **Stanhope and Lancaster's** *Foundations for Population Health in Community/Public Health Nursing*
  - Chapter 14: Disaster Management
- **Stanhope and Lancaster's** *Public Health Nursing*
  - Chapter 21: Public Health Nursing Practice and the Disaster Management Cycle

Case Study Objectives:
After completing this case study, the student should be able to:
1. Describe the essential elements associated with disaster preparation pertinent to older adults at the individual and community level.
2. Identify the applicable elements for a disaster preparation plan for a community-dwelling elder.
3. List major supplies that should be included in a disaster kit for the elderly.
4. Delineate the nurse's role in preparing for a disaster at the personal, professional, and community level.

Disaster Planning and Management Part 2

Response and Recovery

Case Study Synopsis: This case study provides an overview of triage, scene safety, and response. The case study provides assessment of the disaster triage skill set, critical thinking skills, and situational awareness including scene safety.

Estimated Completion Time:
- Case study only: 1 hour
- Plus review questions: + 30 minutes
- Plus discussion questions: + 30 minutes
- Total: 2 hours

Concepts Covered:
- Clinical judgment
- Safety
- Communication
- Care coordination
- Caregiving

Public Health Nursing Interventions Addressed:
- Disease and health event investigation
- Screening
- Collaboration

Suggested Readings:
- **Edelman and Kudzma's** *Health Promotion Throughout the Life Span*
  - Chapter 25: Health Promotion for the Twenty-First Century: Throughout the Lifespan and Throughout the World
- **Nies and McEwen's** *Community/Public Health Nursing*
  - Chapter 29: Natural and Man-Made Disasters
- **Stanhope and Lancaster's** *Foundations for Population Health in Community/Public Health Nursing*
  - Chapter 14: Disaster Management
- **Stanhope and Lancaster's** *Public Health Nursing*
  - Chapter 21: Public Health Nursing Practice and the Disaster Management Cycle

Case Study Objectives:
After completing this case study, the student should be able to:
1. Assess presented scenario for elements of scene safety.
2. Use the principles of triage to prioritize and provide care.
3. Demonstrate immediate care to survivors of disasters.

CASE STUDY 15

Health Literacy

Case Study Synopsis: Martin is a 22-year-old refugee from Uganda who is diagnosed with latent tuberculosis infection (LTBI). He doesn't understand what this means and members of the community fear this is an outbreak brought in by newly arrived refugees. The scenario is about health literacy and not about the LTBI. It is fine if the students have not had the LTBI content.

Estimated Completion Time:
- Case study only: 2 hours
- Plus review questions: + 30 minutes
- Plus discussion questions: + 30 minutes
- Total: 3 hours

Concepts Covered:
- Patient education
- Communication
- Collaboration
- Care coordination

Public Health Nursing Interventions Addressed:
- Advocacy
- Case management
- Surveillance
- Referral and follow-up
- Health education

Suggested Readings:
- **Edelman and Kudzma's *Health Promotion Throughout the Life Span***
  - Chapter 4: The Therapeutic Relationship
  - Chapter 10: Health Education
  - Chapter 11: Nutrition Counseling for Health Promotion

- **Nies and McEwen's *Community/Public Health Nursing***
  - Chapter 1: Health: A Community View
  - Chapter 6: Community Assessment
  - Chapter 8: Community Health Education
- **Stanhope and Lancaster's *Foundations for Population Health in Community/Public Health Nursing***
  - Chapter 11: Using Health Education and Groups in the Community
  - Chapter 12: Community Assessment and Evaluation
- **Stanhope and Lancaster's *Public Health Nursing***
  - Chapter 17: Community as Client: Assessment and Analysis
  - Chapter 19: Health Education Principles Applied in Communities, Groups, Families and Individuals for Healthy Change

Case Study Objectives:
After completing this case study, the student should be able to:
1. Apply health literacy concepts to an individual case study and a community scenario.
2. Interpret readability levels and decide how to use in health education practice.
3. Assess the effectiveness of health teaching at the individual and group level.
4. Synthesize information on cultural awareness and literacy levels at the individual and community level.

Individual Health Promotion

Case Study Synopsis: Teresa is a college health nurse working with a team providing health promotion and disease prevention services for a university community. Using motivational interviewing and the transtheoretical model of change, Teresa is able to work with a college student, Isaiah, and the health promotion topic of sleep.

Estimated Completion Time:
- Case study only: 1 hour
- Plus review questions: + 30 minutes
- Plus discussion questions: + 15 minutes
- Total: 1 hour and 45 minutes

Concepts Covered:
- Health promotion

Public Health Nursing Interventions Addressed:
- Health teaching
- Counseling (motivational interviewing)
- Consultation

Suggested Readings:
- **Edelman and Kudzma's** *Health Promotion Throughout the Life Span*
  - Chapter 1: Health Defined: Objectives for Promotion and Prevention
- **Nies and McEwen's** *Community/Public Health Nursing*
  - Chapter 1: Health: A Community View
  - Chapter 4: Health Promotion and Risk Reduction
- **Stanhope and Lancaster's** *Foundations for Population Health in Community/Public Health Nursing*
  - Chapter 11: Using Health Education and Groups in the Community
- **Stanhope and Lancaster's** *Public Health Nursing*
  - Chapter 18: Building a Culture of Health to Influence Health Equity within Communities
  - Chapter 19: Health Education Principles Applied in Communities, Groups, Families and Individuals for Healthy Change

Case Study Objectives:

After completing this case study, the student should be able to:

1. Differentiate health promotion and disease prevention interventions.
2. Apply motivational interviewing techniques to a member of a community.
3. Incorporate the transtheoretical model of change in providing nursing care to a member of a community.
4. Integrate sleep principles into health promotion care of an individual.

Family Health Promotion

Case Study Synopsis: Nurse Elliott is an RN at an urban based public elementary school in the Midwest. He has been asked to formulate an interprofessional team to provide a community-based health promotion class at the school focusing on preventing obesity.

Estimated Completion Time:
- Case study only: 25 minutes
- Plus review questions: + 20 minutes
- Plus discussion questions: + 15 minutes
- Total: 1 hour

Concepts Covered:
- Leadership
- Health promotion

Public Health Nursing Interventions Addressed:
- Care coordination
- Health teaching
- Health promotion
- Family dynamics

Suggested Readings:
- **Edelman and Kudzma's** *Health Promotion Throughout the Life Span*
  - Unit 2: Emerging Populations and Health
  - Unit 3: Health Policy and the Delivery System
- **Nies and McEwen's** *Community/Public Health Nursing*
  - Chapter 14: Environmental Health
- **Stanhope and Lancaster's** *Foundations for Population Health in Community/Public Health Nursing*
  - Chapter 19: Family Health Risks
- **Stanhope and Lancaster's** *Public Health Nursing*
  - Chapter 19: Health Education Principles Applied in Communities, Groups, Families and Individuals for Healthy Change
  - Chapter 27: Family Health Risks

Case Study Objectives:
After completing this case study, the student should be able to:
1. Describe family-oriented nursing care in the community setting.
2. Utilize collaboration in assessing a problem in the community.
3. Apply health promotion at the community level through patient teaching sessions.

Community Health Promotion

Case Study Synopsis: Clara, RN, BSN, works for the state health department's health promotion division. She is leading an interprofessional coalition to develop a health promotion plan of care to address the opioid crisis in the state.

Estimated Completion Time:
- Case study only: 1 hour
- Plus review questions: + 30 minutes
- Plus discussion questions: + 30 minutes
- Total: 2 hours

Concepts Covered:
- Health promotion

Public Health Nursing Interventions Addressed:
- Coalition building
- Social marketing
- Health education
- Policy development

Suggested Readings:
- **Edelman and Kudzma's** *Health Promotion Throughout the Life Span*
  - Chapter 8: Health Promotion and the Community
- **Nies and McEwen's** *Community/Public Health Nursing*
  - Chapter 1: Health: A Community View
- **Stanhope and Lancaster's** *Foundations for Population Health in Community/Public Health Nursing*
  - Chapter 6: Environmental Health

- Chapter 11: Using Health Education and Groups in the Community
- **Stanhope and Lancaster's** *Public Health Nursing*
  - Chapter 6: Environmental Health
  - Chapter 11: Population-Based Public Health Nursing Practice: The Intervention Wheel
  - Chapter 18: Building a Culture of Health to Influence Health Equity within Communities

Case Study Objectives:
After completing this case study, the student should be able to:
1. Apply an integrated model of health promotion to a health promotion plan of care for a community with an opioid addiction problem.
2. Integrate the nursing process into a health promotion plan of care for a community.
3. Utilize functional health patterns as an assessment framework for evaluating a community.
4. Examine the public health wheel intervention of social marketing.
5. Examine the public health wheel intervention of coalition building.
6. Apply risk communication principles to a plan of care for a community.
7. Integrate the upstream/downstream philosophy of care for a community with an opioid addiction problem.

CASE STUDY 19

Advocating and Working with Diverse Populations

Case Study Synopsis: Community health, experience of care, and economic outcomes can be substantially improved when patients, their families, other caregivers, and the public are fully active participants in care. A military veteran nurse, who is caring for a fellow veteran, advocates for care to assist the client in the management of PTSD.

Estimated Completion Time:
- Case study only: 30 minutes
- Plus review questions: + 20 minutes
- Plus discussion questions: + 10 minutes
- Total: 60 minutes

Concepts Covered:
- Care coordination
- Caregiving
- Stress
- Anxiety
- Addiction
- Culture

Public Health Nursing Interventions Addressed:
- Health promotion
- Advocacy

Suggested Readings:
- **Edelman and Kudzma's** *Health Promotion Throughout the Life Span*
  - Chapter 2: Emerging Populations and Health

- **Nies and McEwen's** *Community/Public Health Nursing*
  - Chapter 22: Veterans' Health
  - Chapter 27: Substance Abuse
- **Stanhope and Lancaster's** *Foundations for Population Health in Community/Public Health Nursing*
  - Chapter 1: Community- and Prevention-Oriented Practice to Improve Population Health
  - Chapter 11: Using Health Education and Groups in the Community
- **Stanhope and Lancaster's** *Public Health Nursing*
  - Chapter 19: Health Education Principles Applied in Communities, Groups, Families and Individuals for Healthy Change
  - Chapter 30: Disability Health Care Across the Lifespan
  - Chapter 36: Mental Health Issues

Case Study Objectives:
After completing this case study, the student should be able to:
1. Describe community-oriented nursing care for veteran populations.
2. Analyze data in assessing a problem in the community.
3. Apply the nursing process at the community level through patient advocacy with diverse populations.

Targeted Health Information for At-Risk Populations

Case Study Synopsis: Nurse Tyra Johnson is an RN at the community health center. She is leading an investigation into the ongoing increase in teenage females that visit the clinic to seek secondary care related to pregnancy.

Estimated Completion Time:
- Case study only: 30 minutes
- Plus review questions: + 20 minutes
- Plus discussion questions: + 10 minutes
- Total: 60 minutes

Concepts Covered:
- Leadership
- Health promotion
- Health policy
- Reproduction

Public Health Nursing Interventions Addressed:
- Surveillance
- Health teaching
- Health promotion

Suggested Readings:
- Edelman and Kudzma's *Health Promotion Throughout the Life Span*
  - Chapter 21: Adolescent
- **Nies and McEwen's** *Community/Public Health Nursing*
  - Chapter 16: Child and Adolescent Health
- **Stanhope and Lancaster's** *Foundations for Population Health in Community/Public Health Nursing*
  - Chapter 1: Community- and Prevention-Oriented Practice to Improve Population Health
- **Stanhope and Lancaster's** *Public Health Nursing*
  - Chapter 1: Public Health Foundations and Population Health
  - Chapter 35: Teen Pregnancy

Case Study Objectives:
After completing this case study, the student should be able to:
1. Prioritize health education information and resources for pregnant teenagers.
2. Analyze data in assessing a problem in the community.
3. Apply the nursing process at the community level through patient teaching sessions.

Evaluate Agency Practices and Policies for Cultural Competence

Case Study Synopsis: George is a clinic manager serving a large Latin American neighborhood. He has a charge of assessing and implementing strategies to make his clinic a more culturally competent place for his population of Latin American people to receive proper care.

Estimated Completion Time:
- Case study only: 1 hour
- Plus review questions: + 30 minutes
- Plus discussion questions: + 30 minutes
- Total: 2 hours

Concepts Covered:
- Culture

Public Health Nursing Interventions Addressed:
- Policy development
- Advocacy
- Collaboration
- Delegated functions

Suggested Readings:
- Nies and McEwen's *Community/Public Health Nursing*
  - Chapter 13: Cultural Diversity and Community Health Nursing
- **Stanhope and Lancaster's** *Foundations for Population Health in Community/Public Health Nursing*
  - Chapter 5: Cultural Influences in Nursing in Community Health
- **Stanhope and Lancaster's** *Public Health Nursing*
  - Chapter 8: Cultural Diversity in the Community

Case Study Objectives:
After completing this case study, the student should be able to:
1. Apply the Campinha-Bacote cultural competence model to individuals and organizations.
2. Assess barriers to cultural competence within organizations.
3. Incorporate a cultural competence model designed for organizations into a health care clinic.
4. Differentiate between cultural competence at clinical, structural, and organizational levels.

CASE STUDY 22

Task Force Development

Case Study Synopsis: Lake Heights has limited access to prescription drug disposal for unused medication. Current disposal methods may be a hazard to water quality. The health department has received limited support in locating a permanent spot to install an unused-prescription medication drop box. Recently a fifth grade student has died from an unintended overdose of her grandmother's unused opioid pain relievers, and the media have reported on the rising rate of heroin addiction in the city. Public health nurse Donita Zwart is charged with the development of a local task force to launch a community unused-prescription medication drop box.

Estimated Completion Time:
- Case study only: 1 hour
- Plus review questions: + 30 minutes
- Plus discussion questions: + 15 minutes
- Total: 1 hour 45 minutes

Concepts Covered:
- Care coordination
- Leadership
- Health promotion
- Health policy

Public Health Nursing Interventions Addressed:
- Outreach
- Health teaching
- Collaboration
- Coalition building
- Community organizing
- Advocacy
- Policy development and enforcement

Suggested Readings:
- Edelman and Kudzma's *Health Promotion Throughout the Life Span*
  - Chapter 1: Health Defined: Health Promotion, Protection, and Prevention
  - Chapter 8: Health Promotion and the Community
- Nies and McEwen's *Community/Public Health Nursing*
  - Chapter 1: Health: A Community View
  - Chapter 3: Thinking Upstream: Nursing Theories and Population-Focused Nursing Practice
  - Chapter 6: Community Assessment
  - Chapter 8: Community Health Education
- Stanhope and Lancaster's *Foundations for Population Health in Community/Public Health Nursing*
  - Chapter 1: Community-Oriented Nursing and Community-Based Nursing
- Stanhope and Lancaster's *Public Health Nursing*
  - Chapter 1: Public Health Foundations and Population Health
  - Chapter 40: The Nurse Leader in the Community

Case Study Objectives:
After completing this case study, the student should be able to:
1. Analyze data in assessing a problem in the community.
2. Apply the nursing process at the community level.
3. Discuss the pros and cons of developing a task force for solving a local community health problem.

Coalition Development

Case Study Synopsis: Public health nurse David became aware last year of a disparity in infant mortality outcomes for African Americans in his county. He is seeking to educate the public about this disparity and discover what can be done. David and his health officer, Linda, worked on a grant recently and were awarded a two-year funding grant to develop education and awareness around this issue in their county's African American community. David will be developing a county-wide coalition to fulfill the grant purpose.

Estimated Completion Time:
- Case study only: 1 hour
- Plus review questions: + 30 minutes
- Plus discussion questions: + 30 minutes
- Total: 2 hours

Concepts Covered:
- Care coordination
- Leadership
- Health promotion
- Health policy

Public Health Nursing Interventions Addressed:
- Outreach
- Health teaching
- Collaboration
- Coalition building
- Community organizing
- Advocacy
- Policy development and enforcement

Suggested Readings:
- **Edelman and Kudzma's** *Health Promotion Throughout the Life Span*
  - Chapter 2: Emerging Populations and Health
  - Chapter 3: Health Policy and the Delivery System
  - Chapter 8: Health Promotion and the Community
- **Nies and McEwen's** *Community/Public Health Nursing*
  - Chapter 7: Community Health Planning, Implementation, and Evaluation
  - Chapter 10: Policy, Politics, Legislation, and Community Health Nursing
- **Stanhope and Lancaster's** *Foundations for Population Health in Community/Public Health Nursing*
  - Chapter 5: Cultural Influences in Nursing in Community Health
  - Chapter 12: Community Assessment and Evaluation
  - Chapter 16: Program Management
- **Stanhope and Lancaster's** *Public Health Nursing*
  - Chapter 1: Public Health Foundations and Population Health
  - Chapter 11: Population-Based Public Health Nursing Practice: The Intervention Wheel
  - Chapter 17: Community as Client: Assessment and Analysis
  - Chapter 18: Building a Culture of Health to Influence Health Equity within Communities

Case Study Objectives:
After completing this case study, the student should be able to:
1. Describe the nursing process in organizing a community coalition.
2. Relate to coalition development within a health planning model.
3. Identify the pros and cons of forming partnerships to promote health improvement.

Navigating the United States Health Care System

Case Study Synopsis: Patient is a 38-year-old Korean female who migrated to the US ten years ago. While performing her monthly breast self-exam she noticed a lump in her left breast. She scheduled an appointment with the local community health clinic for further evaluation.

Estimated Completion Time:
- Case study only: 1 hour
- Plus review questions: + 15 minutes
- Plus discussion questions: + 30 minutes
- Total: 1 hour 45 minutes

Concepts Covered:
- Culture
- Patient education
- Health promotion
- Health care quality

Public Health Nursing Interventions Addressed:
- Screening
- Referral and follow-up
- Case management
- Health teaching

Suggested Readings:
- **Edelman and Kudzma's** *Health Promotion Throughout the Life Span*
  - Chapter 2: Emerging Populations and Health
  - Chapter 9: Screening
  - Chapter 10: Health Education
- **Nies and McEwen's** *Community/Public Health Nursing*
  - Chapter 4: Health Promotion and Risk Reduction
  - Chapter 24: Rural and Migrant Health
- **Stanhope and Lancaster's** *Foundations for Population Health in Community/Public Health Nursing*
  - Chapter 10: Evidence-Based Practice
  - Chapter 11: Using Health Education and Groups in the Community
  - Chapter 20: Health Risks Across the Life Span
- **Stanhope and Lancaster's** *Public Health Nursing*
  - Chapter 10: Evidence-Based Practice
  - Chapter 34: Migrant Health Issues

Case Study Objectives:
After completing this case study, the student should be able to:
1. Demonstrate an understanding of the difference between public and private primary health care entities.
2. Discuss the influence of cost, access, and quality on health care received by the uninsured.
3. Evaluate changes needed in public health and primary care to have an integrated health care delivery system that will improve health outcomes for all people.

CASE STUDY 25

Disease Outbreak
Infectious Disease in a College Dorm

Case Study Synopsis: On January 15, a suspected case of mumps in a student in a college dormitory was reported by student health services. The subsequent investigation uncovered a total of 42 (18 confirmed and 24 probable) more cases of mumps among university students with symptom onset January 13 to April 1.

Estimated Completion Time:
- Case study only: 2 hours
- Plus review questions: + 30 minutes
- Plus discussion questions: + 30 minutes
- Total: 3 hours

Concepts Covered:
- Immunity
- Infection
- Collaboration
- Communication
- Health promotion

Public Health Nursing Interventions Addressed:
- Surveillance
- Disease and health event investigation
- Screening
- Health teaching
- Collaboration

Suggested Readings:
- **Edelman and Kudzma's** *Health Promotion Throughout the Life Span*
  - Chapter 8: Health Promotion and the Community
  - Chapter 9: Screening
  - Chapter 10: Health Education
- **Nies and McEwen's** *Community/Public Health Nursing*
  - Chapter 5: Epidemiology
  - Chapter 8: Community Health Education

- Chapter 26: Communicable Disease
- **Stanhope and Lancaster's** *Foundations for Population Health in Community/Public Health Nursing*
  - Chapter 1: Community and Prevention -Oriented Practices to Improve Population Health
  - Chapter 9: Epidemiological Applications
  - Chapter 11: Using Health Education and Groups in the Community
  - Chapter 15: Surveillance and Outbreak Investigation
  - Chapter 26: Infectious Disease Prevention and Control
  - Chapter 28: Nursing Practice at the Local, State, and National Levels in Public Health
- **Stanhope and Lancaster's** *Public Health Nursing*
  - Chapter 13: Epidemiology
  - Chapter 14: Infectious Disease Prevention and Control
  - Chapter 15: Communicable and Infectious Disease Risks

Case Study Objectives:
After completing this case study, the student should be able to:
1. Discuss trends in the incidence of mumps and identify groups that are at highest risk for infection.
2. Evaluate nursing activities to prevent and control mumps in a community setting.
3. Provide examples of infectious disease control interventions for mumps at the three levels of public health prevention.
4. Describe the public health importance of outbreak investigations.

Disease Outbreak
Foodborne Illness

Case Study Synopsis: Nurse Victoria is an elementary school nurse investigating the sudden increase in gastrointestinal sickness in the Grayson Middle School. Nurse Lydia, the experienced regional public health nurse epidemiologist, works with Victoria to solve the mystery outbreak.

Estimated Completion Time:
- Case study only: 1 hour 30 minutes
- Plus review questions: + 30 minutes
- Plus discussion questions: + 30 minutes
- Total: 2 hours 30 minutes

Concepts Covered:
- Leadership
- Health promotion
- Health policy

Public Health Nursing Interventions Addressed:
- Surveillance
- Disease and health event investigation
- Policy development and enforcement

Suggested Readings:
- Edelman and Kudzma's *Health Promotion Throughout the Life Span*
  - Chapter 9: Screening
  - Chapter 10: Health Education
- Chapter 11: Nutrition Counseling for Health Promotion
- **Nies and McEwen's** *Community/Public Health Nursing*
  - Chapter 5: Epidemiology
  - Chapter 30: School Health
- **Stanhope and Lancaster's** *Foundations for Population Health in Community/Public Health Nursing*
  - Chapter 9: Epidemiological Applications
  - Chapter 20: Health Risks Across the Life Span
  - Chapter 31: The Nurse in the Schools
- **Stanhope and Lancaster's** *Public Health Nursing*
  - Chapter 1: Public Health Foundations and Population Health

Case Study Objectives:
After completing this case study, the student should be able to:
1. Identify ten steps of an outbreak investigation.
2. Describe the six principals of causality.
3. Identify disease onset trends, using an epidemic curve.
4. Apply nursing processes at the community-based level.

Disease Outbreak
Potential Epidemic

Case Study Synopsis: A new nurse infection prevention-ist, Evy Stroup, detects an outbreak of *Clostridium difficile* (*C. difficile*) infection in a hospital. She identifies gaps in infection prevention and works collaboratively with the intensive care unit RN, Josiah Lucas, the infectious dis-ease physician, Dr. Perl, and microbiologist, John Bell, to conduct surveillance to determine infection trends. Evy works to implement prevention measures to halt the outbreak.

Estimated Completion Time:
- Case study only: 2 hours
- Plus review questions: + 30 minutes
- Plus discussion questions: + 15 minutes
- Total: 2 hours 45 minutes

Concepts Covered:
- Leadership
- Health promotion
- Health policy

Public Health Nursing Interventions Addressed:
- Surveillance
- Disease and health event investigation
- Policy development and enforcement

Suggested Readings:

- **Edelman and Kudzma's** *Health Promotion Through-out the Life Span*
  - Chapter 8: Health Promotion and the Community
- **Nies and McEwen's** *Community/Public Health Nursing*
  - Chapter 5: Epidemiology
- **Stanhope and Lancaster's** *Foundations for Popula-tion Health in Community/Public Health Nursing*
  - Chapter 9: Epidemiological Applications
  - Chapter 15. Surveillance and Outbreak Investiga-tion
- **Stanhope and Lancaster's** *Public Health Nursing*
  - Chapter 14: Infectious Disease Prevention and Control

Case Study Objectives:
After completing this case study, the student should be able to:
1. Identify *C. difficile* risk factors.
2. Describe factors associated with infection develop-ment.
3. Identify trends in disease onset.
4. Apply nursing processes at the hospital-based level.

Disease Outbreak
Global Health Risk

Case Study Synopsis: Nurse Rachel is a public health nurse investigating the emerging global health issue involving Zika virus. She is tasked with providing community education and planning a community mosquito eradication plan.

Estimated Completion Time:
- Case study only: 1 hour 30 minutes
- Plus review questions: + 15 minutes
- Plus discussion questions: + 15 minutes
- Total: 2 hours

Concepts Covered:
- Patient education
- Health promotion
- Health policy
- Health disparities

Public Health Nursing Interventions Addressed:
- Disease and other health event investigation
- Outreach
- Health teaching
- Advocacy
- Collaboration
- Coalition building
- Community organizing

Suggested Readings:
- **Edelman and Kudzma's** *Health Promotion Throughout the Life Span*
  - Unit 4: Application of Health Promotion
- Chapter 25: Health Promotion for the 21st Century: Throughout the Life Span and Throughout the World
- **Nies and McEwen's** *Community/Public Health Nursing*
  - Chapter 15: Health in the Global Community
- **Stanhope and Lancaster's** *Foundations for Population Health in Community/Public Health Nursing*
  - Chapter 7: Government, the Law, and Policy Activism
  - Chapter 26: Infectious Disease Prevention and Control
  - Chapter 27: HIV Infection, Hepatitis, Tuberculosis, and Sexually Transmitted Diseases
- **Stanhope and Lancaster's** *Public Health Nursing*
  - Chapter 4: Perspectives in Global Health Care
  - Chapter 14: Infectious Disease Prevention and Control

Case Study Objectives:
After completing this case study, the student should be able to:
1. Discuss the transmission of Zika virus.
2. Identify risk factors for developing Zika virus.
3. Explain the barriers to Zika eradication.
4. List signs, symptoms, and complications of Zika disease.
5. Discuss how lack of funding relates to disparity in terms of Zika virus prevention.

Disease Outbreak
Emerging Disease

Case Study Synopsis: An infection, caused by an emerging infection, carbapenem-resistant Enterobacteriaceae (CRE), a multi drug-resistant bacteria, is identified in three long-term nursing facility residents. The infection prevention and control nurse, Sue Long, works with the department of health to control the outbreak and improve infection prevention measures within the long-term care facility.

Estimated Completion Time:
- Case study only: 1 hour 30 minutes
- Plus review questions: + 15 minutes
- Plus discussion questions: + 15 minutes
- Total: 2 hours

Concepts Covered:
- Leadership
- Health promotion
- Health policy

Public Health Nursing Interventions Addressed:
- Surveillance
- Disease and health event investigation
- Policy development and enforcement

Suggested Readings:
- **Edelman and Kudzma's** *Health Promotion Throughout the Life Span*
  - Chapter 8: Health Promotion and the Community
- **Nies and McEwen's** *Community/Public Health Nursing*
  - Chapter 5: Epidemiology
- **Stanhope and Lancaster's** *Foundations for Population Health in Community/Public Health Nursing*
  - Chapter 9: Epidemiological Applications
  - Chapter 15: Surveillance and Outbreak Investigation
- **Stanhope and Lancaster's** *Public Health Nursing*
  - Chapter 14: Infectious Disease Prevention and Control

Case Study Objectives:
After completing this case study, the student should be able to:
1. Identify the characteristics of carbapenem-resistant Enterobacteriaceae (CRE).
2. Describe risk factors for developing CRE.
3. Apply nursing processes to improve infection prevention and control.

Community-Based Participatory Research

Case Study Synopsis: Pat is an RN manager of a veteran's health administration (VHA) community-based outreach clinic (CBOC) associated with a large urban tertiary medical center. The strategic plan charges five regional CBOC managers to evaluate their clinics' health services provided to the veterans living in their community to ensure excellence in healthy outcomes as identified by strategic plan outcome metrics.

Estimated Completion Time:
- Case study only: 3 hours
- Plus review questions: + 30 minutes
- Plus discussion questions: + 45 minutes
- Total: 4 hours 15 minutes

Concepts Covered:
- Leadership
- Health promotion
- Health policy

Public Health Nursing Interventions Addressed:
- Surveillance
- Health teaching
- Advocacy
- Outreach
- Screening

Suggested Readings:
- **Edelman and Kudzma's** *Health Promotion Throughout the Life Span*
  - Chapter 8: Health Promotion and the Community
- **Nies and McEwen's** *Community/Public Health Nursing*
  - Chapter 8: Community Health Education
  - Chapter 22: Veterans' Health
- **Stanhope and Lancaster's** *Foundations for Population Health in Community/Public Health Nursing*
  - Chapter 9: Epidemiological Applications
- **Stanhope and Lancaster's** *Public Health Nursing*
  - Chapter 18: Building a Culture of Health to Influence Health Equity within Communities
  - Chapter 20: The Nurse-Managed Health Center: A Model for Public Health Nursing Practice
  - Chapter 24: Quality Management

Case Study Objectives:
After completing this case study, the student should be able to:
1. Locate sources for an identified population's demographic and health status data.
2. Create a plan to involve stakeholders in addressing community health concerns.
3. Understand how Photovoice is used in community-based participatory research (CBPR).
4. Identify a CBPR plan.
5. Become familiar with a variety of models to evaluate the CBPR outcomes.

CASE STUDY 31

Board of Health Report

Case Study Synopsis: Public health nurse Tammie sharpens her communication and team-leading skills in heading up the effort to report key public health activities to the local board of health.

Estimated Completion Time:
- Case study only: 1 hour
- Plus review questions: + 15 minutes
- Plus discussion questions: + 30 minutes
- Total: 1 hour 45 minutes

Concepts Covered:
- Leadership
- Health policy
- Health care organizations
- Health care economics

Public Health Nursing Interventions Addressed:
- Delegated functions
- Health teaching
- Consultation
- Advocacy
- Policy development

Suggested Readings:
- **Edelman and Kudzma's** *Health Promotion Throughout the Life Span*
  - Chapter 3: Health Policy and the Delivery System
  - Chapter 8: Health Promotion and the Community

- **Nies and McEwen's** *Community/Public Health Nursing*
  - Chapter 1: Health: A Community View
  - Chapter 10: Policy, Politics, Legislation and Community Health Nursing
- **Stanhope and Lancaster's** *Foundations for Population Health in Community/Public Health Nursing*
  - Chapter 1: Community- and Prevention-Oriented Practice to Improve Population Health
- **Stanhope and Lancaster's** *Public Health Nursing*
  - Chapter 24: Quality Management
  - Chapter 40: The Nurse Leader in the Community
  - Chapter 46: Public Health Nursing at Local, State, and National Levels

Case Study Objectives:
After completing this case study, the student should be able to:
1. Identify sources of funding for public health agencies.
2. Describe the impact that various funding sources have on individuals and services available in the community.
3. Relate the impact that informatics in nursing has on reporting service activities to key stakeholders in public health.

Proposal for Funding from External Source

Case Study Synopsis: A nursing class plans and implements an organ donation awareness campaign with funding from a state public health department grant.

Estimated Completion Time:
- Case study only: 30 minutes
- Plus review questions: + 15 minutes
- Plus discussion questions: + 15 minutes
- Total: 1 hour

Concepts Covered:
- Health care economics

Public Health Interventions Addressed:
- Social marketing
- Health teaching
- Community organizing

Suggested Readings:
- **Nies and McEwen's** *Community/Public Health Nursing*
  - Chapter 7: Community Health Planning, Implementation, and Evaluation
  - Chapter 12: Economics of Health Care

- **Stanhope and Lancaster's** *Foundations for Population Health in Community/Public Health Nursing*
  - Chapter 8: Economic Influences
  - Chapter 16: Program Management
- **Stanhope and Lancaster's** *Public Health Nursing*
  - Chapter 5: Economics of Healthcare Delivery
  - Chapter 23: Program Management

Case Study Objectives:
After completing this case study, the student should be able to:
1. Identify the steps in the health planning model.
2. Differentiate between cognitive, affective, and psychomotor learning domains.
3. Recognize the role of the nurse in program management.
4. Identify levels of prevention in program planning and evaluation.
5. Identify the role of social marketing in program management.
6. Understand the role of grant funding in health promotion.

Delivering Care within Budgetary Guidelines

Case Study Synopsis: Nurse Brown, a manager at a rural health department, works with community partners to improve influenza vaccination rates. She leads the community wide effort and must make several decisions regarding the community size, targeted population, and her allocated budget.

Estimated Completion Time:
- Case study only: 1 hour
- Plus review questions: + 30 minutes
- Plus discussion questions: + 30 minutes
- Total: 2 hours

Concepts Covered:
- Patient education
- Health promotion
- Communication
- Collaboration
- Health disparities
- Health care economics

Public Health Nursing Interventions Addressed:
- Collaboration
- Community organization and building
- Advocacy
- Health teaching

Suggested Readings:

- **Nies and McEwen's** *Community/Public Health Nursing*
  - Chapter 12: Economics of Health Care
- **Stanhope and Lancaster's** *Foundations for Population Health in Community/Public Health Nursing*
  - Chapter 8: Economic Influences
- **Stanhope and Lancaster's** *Public Health Nursing*
  - Chapter 5: Economics of Health Care Delivery
  - Chapter 14: Infectious Disease Prevention and Control
  - Chapter 40: The Nurse Leader in the Community

Case Study Objectives:
After completing this case study, the student should be able to:
1. Determine costs of planning a public health flu shot project.
2. Justify eliminating some clinics based on a cost analysis.
3. Make decisions based on community needs and budgetary limitations.
4. Plan and budget flu prevention programs that will serve targeted populations.
5. Solicit financial support from community agencies that will contribute to the community's overall health.

Conflict Resolution

Case Study Synopsis: Nurse Lisa is a public health nurse in a community center for low-income residents. Her manager has directed her to work with the residents to solve ongoing conflicts between many of them. In addressing the need for conflict resolution education, nurse Lisa will teach the residents how to follow the chain of command when there is conflict in the community center, as well as in their own day-to-day activities.

Estimated Completion Time:
- Case study only: 1 hour
- Plus review questions: + 30 minutes
- Plus discussion questions: + 15 minutes
- Total: 1 hour 45 minutes

Concepts Covered:
- Leadership
- Communication
- Interpersonal violence

Public Health Nursing Interventions Addressed:
- Surveillance
- Advocacy
- Health teaching
- Nursing process

Suggested Readings:
- **Edelman and Kudzma's** *Health Promotion Throughout the Life Span*
  - Chapter 4: The Therapeutic Relationship
  - Chapter 8: Health Promotion and the Community
- **Nies and McEwen's** *Community/Public Health Nursing*
  - Chapter 3: Thinking Upstream: Nursing Theories and Population-Focused Nursing Practice
- **Stanhope and Lancaster's** *Foundations for Population Health in Community/Public Health Nursing*
  - Chapter 11: Using Health Education and Groups in the Community
  - Chapter 13: Case Management
  - Chapter 21: Vulnerability and Vulnerable Populations: An Overview
  - Chapter 25: Violence and Human Abuse
- **Stanhope and Lancaster's** *Public Health Nursing*
  - Chapter 1: Public Health Foundations and Population Health
  - Chapter 16: Promoting Healthy Communities
  - Chapter 25: Case Management
  - Chapter 40: The Nurse Leader in the Community

Case Study Objectives:

After completing this case study, the student should be able to:

1. Apply the nursing process to conflict resolution.
2. Identify interpersonal violence in vulnerable populations.
3. Apply leadership skills and chain-of-command education.
4. Define conflict and conflict resolution.
5. Understand the role of the case manager in conflict resolution in public health communities.

CASE STUDY 35

Adhering to Ethical Standards

Case Study Synopsis: Morgan is a public health nurse who has just begun employment at the free community health care clinic. This clinic serves homeless adults, teenagers, and families with small children. Several agencies also provide services in the same building to better serve this marginalized population.

Estimated Completion Time:
- Case study only: 2 hours
- Plus review questions: + 30 minutes
- Plus discussion questions: + 30 minutes
- Total: 3 hours

Concepts Covered:
- Leadership
- Ethics
- Health promotion
- Collaboration
- Health policy
- Health care law

Public Health Nursing Interventions Addressed:
- Health teaching
- Advocacy
- Outreach
- Screening

Suggested Readings:
- **Edelman and Kudzma's** *Health Promotion Throughout the Life Span*
  - Chapter 5: Ethical Issues Related to Health Promotion
  - Chapter 9: Screening

- Chapter 10: Health Education
- **Nies and McEwen's** *Community/Public Health Nursing*
  - Chapter 16: Child and Adolescent Health
- **Stanhope and** *Lancaster's Foundations for Population Health in Community/Public Health Nursing*
  - Chapter 4: Ethics in Public Health and Community Health Nursing Practice
  - Chapter 20: Health Risks Across the Lifespan
  - Chapter 29: The Faith Community Nurse
- **Stanhope and Lancaster's** *Public Health Nursing*
  - Chapter 7: Application of Ethics in the Community
  - Chapter 25: Case Management

Case Study Objectives:
After completing this case study, the student should be able to:
1. Determine the relationship of ethical theories to the public health nurse's role in health care delivery and health promotion.
2. Discuss the similarities and differences between the nursing code of ethics and the public health nursing code of ethics.
3. Assess present public health ethical issues in health care delivery and health promotion in community-based nursing.
4. Analyze public health issues related to ethical decision-making.

Nurse-Managed Centers

Case Study Synopsis: Registered nurse Carol and nurse practitioner Cheryl are planning to be partners in a community-based nurse-managed center that provides services to populations across their lifespans.

Estimated Completion Time:

- Case study only: 1 hour
- Plus review questions: + 20 minutes
- Plus discussion questions: + 30 minutes
- Total: 1 hour 50 minutes

Concepts Covered:

- Professional identity
- Clinical judgment
- Leadership
- Patient education
- Health promotion
- Collaboration
- Evidence
- Health care quality
- Health disparities

Public Health Nursing Interventions Addressed:

- Advocacy
- Collaboration
- Case management
- Consultation
- Counseling
- Disease investigation
- Outreach
- Referral and follow-up
- Screening

Suggested Readings:

- **Edelman and Kudzma's** *Health Promotion Throughout the Life Span*
  - Chapter 3: Health Policy and the Delivery System
- **Nies & McEwen's** *Community/Public Health Nursing*
  - Chaper 12: Economics of Health Care
- **Stanhope and Lancaster's** *Foundations for Population Health in Community/Public Health Nursing*
  - Chapter 8: Economic Influences
- **Stanhope and Lancaster's** *Public Health Nursing*
  - Chapter 5: Economics of Health Care Delivery
  - Chapter 20: The Nurse-Managed Health Center: A Model for Public Health Nursing Practice

Case Study Objectives:

After completing this case study, the student should be able to:

1. Describe the key characteristics of a nurse-managed center.
2. Differentiate the responsibilities of the registered nurse and the nurse practitioner in nurse-managed centers.
3. Discuss the importance of evidence-based practice in a community-based center.
4. Explain the importance of community collaboration in building a successful nurse-managed center.

Quality Management and Improvement

Case Study Synopsis: Casey is a cancer detection specialist nurse who is assigned the task of identifying and implementing a quality improvement project to address the low completion rates for patients referred for colorectal cancer screening.

Estimated Completion Time:
- Case study only: 2 hours
- Plus review questions: + 30 minutes
- Plus discussion questions: + 2 hours
- Total: 4 hours 30 minutes

Concepts Covered:
- Leadership
- Health promotion
- Health care quality

Public Health Nursing Interventions Addressed:
- Referral and follow-up
- Health teaching
- Counseling
- Social marketing
- Outreach

Suggested Readings:
- **Edelman and Kudzma's** *Health Promotion Throughout the Life Span*
  - Chapter 3: Health Policy and the Delivery System
- **Nies and McEwen's** *Community/Public Health Nursing*
  - Chapter 11: The Health Care System
- **Stanhope and Lancaster's** *Foundations for Population Health in Community/Public Health Nursing*
  - Chapter 17: Managing Quality and Safety
- **Stanhope and Lancaster's** *Public Health Nursing*
  - Chapter 24: Quality Management

Case Study Objectives:
After completing this case study, the student should be able to:
1. Differentiate between scientific research and program evaluation research.
2. Identify quality indicators for a specific health prevention program.
3. Apply a quality improvement process to a community clinic.
4. Determine specific outcomes of quality improvement projects.
5. Use Plan-Do-Study-Act cycles as a program evaluation tool.

Public Health Workforce

Case Study Synopsis: ABC Hospital is applying for Magnet status. The board of directors has met to discuss how this can be accomplished. One suggestion is to increase their contribution to the community, and an idea to build a community health clinic is proposed. One of the hospital's public health nurses (PHN) is asked to plan a community health clinic. The planning involves hiring a workforce, and the PHN is using the Quad Council Coalition Competency Review Task Force and the US Public Health Service competency guidelines to identify requirements for qualified staff.

Estimated Completion Time:
- Case study only: 1 hour
- Plus review questions: + 30 minutes
- Plus discussion questions: + 15 minutes
- Total: 1 hour 45 minutes

Concepts Covered:
- Leadership

Public Health Nursing Interventions Addressed:
- Professional development
- Team work
- Leadership
- Communication

Suggested Readings:
- **Stanhope and Lancaster's** *Foundations for Population Health in Community/Public Health Nursing*
  - Chapter 1: Community- and Prevention-Oriented Practice to Improve Population Health
  - Chapter 3: The Changing U.S. Health and Public Health Care Systems
- **Stanhope and Lancaster's** *Public Health Nursing*
  - Chapter 1: Public Health Foundations and Population Health
  - Chapter 7: Application of Ethics in the Community
  - Chapter 23: Program Management
  - Chapter 40: The Nurse Leader in the Community
  - Chapter 46: Public Health Nursing at Local, State, and National Levels

Case Study Objectives:
After completing this case study, the student should be able to:
1. Explore the various nursing education levels, continuing education, and professional development opportunities in public health nursing.
2. Identify competencies required of a public health nurse based on the public health core functions.
3. Examine the roles of various levels of nursing in the public health workforce.
4. Evaluate public health workforce and practices.
5. Implement leadership skills within the public health workforce.

CASE STUDY 39

Populations Affected with Disabilities

Case Study Synopsis: Clients in rural areas tend to have a poor understanding of their health and functional status. Older clients are less likely to practice preventive health care and more likely to smoke, use alcohol, and be obese. A 76-year-old disabled Hispanic male, who has been a client of the public health service for three years, is visited by a public health nurse.

Estimated Completion Time:
- Case study only: 3 hours
- Plus review questions: + 30 minutes
- Plus discussion questions: + 30 minutes
- Total: 4 hours

Concepts Covered:
- Functional ability
- Adherence
- Glucose regulation
- Nutrition
- Gas exchange
- Mobility
- Sensory perception
- Addiction
- Patient education
- Care coordination

Public Health Nursing Interventions Addressed:
- Outreach
- Case finding
- Referral and follow-up
- Case management
- Delegated functions
- Health teaching
- Counseling
- Consultation
- Advocacy

Suggested Readings:
- **Edelman and Kudzma's** *Health Promotion Throughout the Life Span*
  - Chapter 3: Health Policy and the Delivery System
- **Nies and McEwen's** *Community/Public Health Nursing*
  - Chapter 21: Populations Affected by Disabilities
- **Stanhope and Lancaster's** *Foundations for Population Health in Community/Public Health Nursing*
  - Chapter 21: Vulnerability and Vulnerable Populations: An Overview
  - Chapter 24: Alcohol, Tobacco, and Other Drug Problems in the Community
- **Stanhope and Lancaster's** *Public Health Nursing*
  - Chapter 30: Disability Health Care Across the Life Span

Case Study Objectives:
After completing this case study, the student should be able to:
1. Differentiate between the purposes, benefits, and limitations of government-sponsored programs for those members who are disabled to achieve health equity.
2. Describe attitudes and perceptions that contribute to the treatment of people with disabilities.
3. Identify health care and social issues that influence people with disabilities.
4. Promote the health and well-being of people with disabilities.
5. Explain the role of the nurse in providing primary, secondary, and tertiary prevention of alcohol and tobacco abuse.
6. Discuss the impact of substance abuse on clients in a community.
7. Describe factors that may lead to disabilities in certain populations.
8. Examine how public policies reduce health disparities for people with disabilities.
9. Discuss strategies that public health nurses may use to improve the health status of people with disabilities.

Poverty and Homelessness

Case Study Synopsis: Public health nurse David assists people who are homeless in his community.

Estimated Completion Time:
- Case study only: 1 hour
- Plus review questions: + 30 minutes
- Plus discussion questions: + 30 minutes
- Total: 2 hours

Concepts Covered:
- Coping
- Clinical judgement
- Leadership
- Health promotion
- Communication
- Collaboration
- Safety
- Care coordination
- Health disparities

Public Health Nursing Interventions Addressed:
- Surveillance
- Disease and health event investigation
- Outreach
- Screening
- Referral and follow-up
- Case management
- Collaboration
- Advocacy

Suggested Readings:
- **Edelman and Kudzma's** *Health Promotion Throughout the Life Span*
  - Chapter 2: Emerging Populations and Health
- **Nies and McEwen's** *Community/Public Health Nursing*
  - Chapter 23: Homeless Populations
- **Stanhope and Lancaster's** *Foundations for Population Health in Community/Public Health Nursing*
  - Chapter 23: Poverty, Homelessness, Teen Pregnancy, and Mental Illness
- **Stanhope and Lancaster's** *Public Health Nursing*
  - Chapter 33: Poverty and Homelessness

Case Study Objectives:

After completing this case study, the student should be able to:

1. Analyze factors that contribute to risk of homelessness.
2. Identify and prioritize nursing interventions for populations who are homeless.
3. Discuss the effects of poverty on health and well-being.
4. Identify resources at federal, state, and local levels that address homelessness.

Rural and Migrant Health

Case Study Synopsis: Nurse Lexi is a public health nurse working with Hispanic migrant farm families in camps and the work site. Fifteen of the migrant workers have been diagnosed with tuberculosis.

Estimated Completion Time:
- Case study only: 1 hour
- Plus review questions: + 15 minutes
- Plus discussion questions: + 15 minutes
- Total: 1 hour 30 minutes

Concepts Covered:
- Culture
- Spirituality
- Immunity
- Infection
- Clinical judgment
- Leadership
- Patient education
- Health promotion
- Health disparities

Public Health Nursing Interventions Addressed:
- Surveillance
- Screening
- Health teaching
- Collaboration

Suggested Readings:
- **Nies and McEwen's** *Community/Public Health Nursing*
  - Chapter 13: Cultural Diversity and Community Health Nursing
- Chapter 24: Rural and Migrant Health
- Chapter 26: Communicable Diseases
- **Stanhope and Lancaster's** *Foundations for Population Health in Community/Public Health Nursing*
  - Chapter 5: Cultural Influences in Nursing in Community Health
  - Chapter 9: Epidemiological Applications
  - Chapter 15: Surveillance and Outbreak Investigation
  - Chapter 22: Rural Health and Migrant Health
- **Stanhope and Lancaster's** *Public Health Nursing*
  - Chapter 8: Cultural Diversity in the Community
  - Chapter 15: Communicable and Infectious Disease Risks
  - Chapter 22: Public Health Surveillance and Outbreak Investigation
  - Chapter 34: Migrant Health Issues

Case Study Objectives:
After completing this case study, the student should be able to:
1. Analyze behaviors of Hispanic migrant workers that put them at risk for tuberculosis.
2. Identify the role of the public health nurse in surveillance and outbreak investigation when working with tuberculosis.
3. Analyze the role of the public health nurse in planning and implementing culturally competent care for Hispanic migrant workers.

Substance Abuse

Case Study Synopsis: A public health nurse working in a substance abuse recovery clinic examines one client's struggle with addiction and community efforts to address substance abuse.

Estimated Completion Time:
- Case study only: 1 hour
- Plus review questions: + 30 minutes
- Plus discussion questions: + 30 minutes
- Total: 2 hours

Concepts Covered:
- Addiction
- Patient education
- Health promotion

Public Health Nursing Interventions Addressed:
- Health teaching
- Counseling
- Outreach

Suggested Readings:
- Edelman and Kudzma's *Health Promotion Throughout the Life Span*
  - Chapter 21: Adolescent
- **Nies and McEwen's** *Community/Public Health Nursing*
  - Chapter 27: Substance Abuse
- **Stanhope and Lancaster's** *Foundations for Population Health in Community/Public Health Nursing*
  - Chapter 24: Alcohol, Tobacco, and Other Drug Problems in the Community
- **Stanhope and Lancaster's** *Public Health Nursing*
  - Chapter 37: Alcohol, Tobacco, and Other Drug Problems

Case Study Objectives:
After completing this case study, the student should be able to:
1. Identify potential behaviors associated with addiction.
2. Describe the 12 steps used in recovery from alcohol and narcotic abuse.
3. Discuss the nurse's role in preventing and addressing addiction at the individual and community levels.

Violence and Human Abuse

Case Study Synopsis: School nurse Nancy discovers a student who is the victim of abuse and has witnessed significant violence in her home. She works through the referral process with Aaron, a nursing student.

Estimated Completion Time:
- Case study only: 30 minutes
- Plus review questions: + 15 minutes
- Plus discussion questions: + 30 minutes
- Total: 1 hour 15 minutes

Concepts Covered:
- Family dynamics
- Sleep
- Pain
- Stress
- Coping
- Addiction
- Interpersonal violence
- Clinical judgment
- Health disparities

Public Health Nursing Interventions Addressed:
- Disease and health event investigation
- Collaboration
- Advocacy
- Referral and follow-up
- Counseling

Suggested Readings:
- **Edelman and Kudzma's** *Health Promotion Throughout the Life Span*
  - Chapter 4: The Therapeutic Relationship
- **Nies and McEwen's** *Community/Public Health Nursing*
  - Chapter 24: Rural and Migrant Health
  - Chapter 30: School Health
- **Stanhope and Lancaster's** *Foundations for Population Health in Community/Public Health Nursing*
  - Chapter 24: Alcohol, Tobacco, and Other Drug Problems in the Community
  - Chapter 25: Violence and Human Abuse
- **Stanhope and Lancaster's** *Public Health Nursing*
  - Chapter 27: Family Health Risks

Case Study Objectives:
After completing this case study, the student should be able to:
1. Discuss public health strategies for preventing violence and its consequences.
2. Apply the nursing process in the identification and screening of child maltreatment.
3. Define three factors that influence violence and human abuse.

CASE STUDY 44

Case Management

Case Study Synopsis: Karen, a county public health nurse, is called by a clinic to assist a local family. Cora is pregnant with her second child, and the first pregnancy ended in the stillbirth of her baby girl. Cora's physician is concerned that Cora has started prenatal care at 16 weeks, and now has missed her next appointment. He knows that she needs to have access to resources in the community to support her health, and has referred her case to the public health department for case management.

Estimated Completion Time:
- Case study only: 1 hour
- Plus review questions: + 30 minutes
- Plus discussion questions: + 15 minutes
- Total: 1 hour 45 minutes

Concepts Covered:
- Family dynamics
- Culture
- Adherence
- Collaboration
- Care coordination

Public Health Nursing Interventions Addressed:
- Referral and follow-up
- Case management
- Health teaching
- Consultation
- Collaboration
- Advocacy

Suggested Readings:
- **Edelman and Kudzma's** *Health Promotion Throughout the Life Span*
  - Chapter 3: Health Policy and the Delivery System
- **Nies and McEwen's** *Community/Public Health Nursing*
  - Chapter 4: Health Promotion and Risk Reduction
  - Chapter 13: Cultural Diversity and Community Health Nursing
- **Stanhope and Lancaster's** *Foundations for Population Health in Community/Public Health Nursing*
  - Chapter 5: Cultural Influences in Nursing in Community Health
  - Chapter 13: Case Management
- **Stanhope and Lancaster's** *Public Health Nursing*
  - Chapter 8: Cultural Diversity in the Community
  - Chapter 11: Population-Based Public Health Nursing Practice: The Intervention Wheel
  - Chapter 25: Case Management

Case Study Objectives:
After completing this case study, the student should be able to:
1. Compare and contrast the role of nurse case manager and care coordinator.
2. Describe the scope of practice of the nurse case manager in the given scenario.
3. Apply the nursing process at the case manager level.
4. Discuss the value of culturally congruent care in the delivery of case management services.

Faith Community Nursing

Case Study Synopsis: A nurse researches faith community nursing and what is involved in being a faith community nurse.

Estimated Completion Time:
- Case study only: 2 hours
- Plus review questions: + 30 minutes
- Plus discussion questions: + 1 hour 30 minutes
- Total: 4 hours

Concepts Covered:
- Health care organizations
- Culture

Public Health Nursing Interventions Addressed:
- Health teaching
- Advocacy
- Counseling
- Surveillance
- Referral and follow-up
- Community organizing

Suggested Readings:
- **Edelman and Kudzma's** *Health Promotion Throughout the Life Span*
  - Chapter 13: Stress Management
- **Nies and McEwen's** *Community/Public Health Nursing*
  - Chapter 33: Faith Community Nursing
- **Stanhope and Lancaster's** *Foundations for Population Health in Community/Public Health Nursing*
  - Chapter 29: The Faith Community Nurse
- **Stanhope and Lancaster's** *Public Health Nursing*
  - Chapter 45: The Nurse in the Faith Community

Case Study Objectives:

After completing this case study, the student should be able to:

1. Define faith community nursing.
2. Discuss healing ministries.
3. Compare public health issues with the development of faith community nursing.
4. Evaluate faith community nursing models as they relate to the scope and practice of faith community nursing.
5. Identify the nurse's role in providing spiritual care, health promotion, and disease prevention in faith communities.
6. Compare and contrast spirituality and religiosity.

Forensic and Correctional Nursing

Case Study Synopsis: Nurse Kaitlyn is a sexual assault nurse examiner (SANE) who works with a correctional facility and the forensic department in her community. She is working with a 16-year-old female who has been raped, does not remember what happened, and is accompanied by a male person who is not a family member who will not leave her side.

Estimated Completion Time:
- Case study only: 1 hour
- Plus review questions + 15 minutes
- Plus discussion questions: + 15 minutes
- Total: 1 hour 30 minutes

Concepts Covered:
- Sexuality
- Stress
- Mood and affect
- Anxiety
- Clinical judgment
- Leadership
- Ethics
- Patient education
- Communication
- Collaboration
- Safety
- Care coordination
- Health care law

Public Health Nursing Interventions Addressed:
- Disease and health event investigation
- Referral and follow-up
- Case management
- Health teaching
- Counseling
- Collaboration
- Policy development and enforcement

Suggested Readings:
- **Nies and McEwen's** *Community/Public Health Nursing*
  - Chapter 28: Violence
  - Chapter 32: Forensic and Correctional Nursing
- **Stanhope and Lancaster's** *Foundations for Population Health in Community/Public Health Nursing*
  - Chapter 25: Violence and Human Abuse
- **Stanhope and Lancaster's** *Public Health Nursing*
  - Chapter 38: Violence and Human Abuse
  - Chapter 44: Forensic Nursing in the Community

Case Study Objectives:
After completing this case study, the student should be able to:
1. Identify three factors that influence violence and human abuse.
2. Implement nursing interventions for populations who are victims of sexual abuse/rape/human trafficking.
3. Identify competencies and skills for the forensic nurse and the SANE in practice.
4. Implement nursing interventions that relate to the three levels of prevention employed by the forensic nurse and the SANE.
5. Collaborate with other health care team members, police, and others in the community to address prevention of sexual abuse/rape/human trafficking.

Genomics

Case Study Synopsis: Nurse Leslie is admitting a new patient to the primary care setting and needs to assess for health promotion and disease prevention links to genetics and genomics.

Estimated Completion Time:
- Case study only: 1 hour
- Plus review questions: + 30 minutes
- Plus discussion questions: + 30 minutes
- Total: 2 hours

Concepts Covered:
- Stress and coping
- Ethics
- Health promotion
- Patient education
- Technology
- Communication
- Evidence
- Health care quality
- Health disparities
- Health care law

Public Health Nursing Interventions Addressed:
- Consultation
- Counseling
- Health teaching
- Referral and follow-up
- Screening

Suggested Readings:
- **Stanhope and Lancaster's** *Public Health Nursing*
  - Chapter 12: Genomics in Public Health Nursing

Case Study Objectives:

After completing this case study, the student should be able to:

1. Articulate skills and strengths nurses need to acquire to complement the work of other health care providers to improve the health of the public.
2. Cultivate communication skills to assess an individual, family, and community for risk of developing disease and opportunities for health promotion.
3. Consider how social determinants of health have influenced health disparities and health care law.
4. Articulate the relationship between ethical information exchange in patient education and the role this plays in health promotion of the individual, family, and/or community.
5. Describe the changing technological processes for screening and evidence for use of genetics and genomics to promote quality community health care.
6. Explain how identifying resilience in an individual, family, and/or community can reduce stress and increase coping during genetics/genomics assessment.

CASE STUDY 48

Global Health

Case Study Synopsis: A public health nurse leads an interdisciplinary nongovernmental organization (NGO) called SALUD. This NGO is looking to begin a long-term, mutually beneficial engagement with a community in Central America and an academic institution in the United States. This case unfolds over years as the public health nurse guides the group through the public health process, laying a strong foundation with a thorough assessment and development of engaged, long-term community partnerships. The team eventually decides on five priority health areas, and continues to plan and develop interventions and evaluation methods to improve the health of the local population.

Estimated Completion Time:

- Case study only: 2 hours
- Plus review questions: + 30 minutes
- Plus discussion questions: + 30 minutes
- Total: 3 hours

Concepts Covered:

- Health disparities
- Collaboration
- Clinical judgment
- Leadership
- Ethics
- Health promotion
- Culture
- Stress

Public Health Nursing Interventions Addressed:

- Surveillance
- Collaboration
- Community organization building
- Advocacy
- Policy development

Suggested Readings:

- **Edelman and Kudzma's** *Health Promotion Throughout the Life Span*
  - Chapter 25: Health Promotion for the Twenty-First Century: Throughout the Life Span and Throughout the World

- **Nies and McEwen's** *Community/Public Health Nursing*
  - Chapter 1: Health: A Community View
  - Chapter 3: Thinking Upstream: Nursing Theories and Population-Focused Nursing Practice
  - Chapter 5: Epidemiology
  - Chapter 6: Community Assessment
  - Chapter 7: Community Health Planning, Implementation, and Evaluation
  - Chapter 15: Health in the Global Community
  - Chapter 20: Family Health
- **Stanhope and Lancaster's** *Foundations for Population Health in Community/Public Health Nursing*
  - Chapter 1: Community and Prevention-Oriented Practice to Improve Population Health
  - Chapter 16: Program Management
  - Chapter 25: Violence and Human Abuse
- **Stanhope and Lancaster's** *Public Health Nursing*
  - Chapter 1: Public Health Foundations and Population Health
  - Chapter 4: Perspectives in Global Health Care
  - Chapter 11: Population-Based Public Health Nursing Practice: The Intervention Wheel
  - Chapter 17: Building a Culture of Health to Influence Health Equity within Communities
  - Chapter 23: Program Management
  - Chapter 38: Violence and Human Abuse

Case Study Objectives:

After completing this case study, the student should be able to:

1. Describe the process of conducting a community health assessment, detailing the challenges faced in the global environment.
2. Utilize the International Community Assessment Model (ICAM) as a guide for initial assessment.
3. Utilize epidemiologic and demographic data as part of the assessment process.

Home Health and Hospice

Case Study Synopsis: A 56-year-old male who lives in a rural area of Kentucky with his sister is referred to hospice for end-stage heart disease. The hospital discharge planner shares that there is a known history of opioid abuse in the home environment.

Estimated Completion Time:
- Case study only: 2 hours
- Plus review questions: + 30 minutes
- Plus discussion questions: + 30 minutes
- Total: 3 hours

Concepts Covered:
- Patient education
- Pain
- Stress
- Coping
- Nutrition

Public Health Nursing Interventions Addressed:
- Policy development and enforcement
- Collaboration
- Health teaching
- Case management

Suggested Readings:
- **Edelman and Kudzma's** *Health Promotion Throughout the Life Span*
  - Chapter 4: The Therapeutic Relationship
  - Chapter 24: Older Adult
- **Nies and McEwen's** *Community/Public Health Nursing*
  - Chapter 24: Rural and Migrant Health
  - Chapter 27: Substance Abuse
  - Chapter 34: Home Health and Hospice
- **Stanhope and Lancaster's** *Foundations for Population Health in Community/Public Health Nursing*
  - Chapter 24: Alcohol, Tobacco, and Other Drug Problems in the Community
  - Chapter 30: The Nurse in Home Health and Hospice
- **Stanhope and Lancaster's** *Public Health Nursing*
  - Chapter 37: Alcohol, Tobacco, and Other Drug Problems
  - Chapter 41: The Nurse in Home Health, Palliative Care, and Hospice

Case Study Objectives:
After completing this case study, the student should be able to:
1. Identify and predict the challenges for pain management in a home environment with substance abuse.
2. Design a care plan to offer pain and symptom management for a patient with comorbidities (end-stage heart disease, malnutrition, and pain).
3. Compare and contrast the needs of the patient in an inpatient hospice setting versus the patient's home setting.
4. Identify strategies to support the emotional needs of the patient and family members during the terminal phase of life.

Occupational Health

Case Study Synopsis: Casey, who is an occupational and environmental health nurse (OHN), works the day shift at a meat packing plant. There are 500 employees on the day shift and 350 on the evening shift, in addition to administrators, ancillary personnel, and office staff.

Estimated Completion Time:
- Case study only: 3 hours
- Plus review questions: + 1 hour
- Plus discussion questions: + 3 hours
- Total: 7 hours

Concepts Covered:
- Professionalism
- Leadership
- Patient education
- Health promotion
- Communication
- Health care quality

Public Health Nursing Interventions Addressed:
- Health teaching
- Counseling
- Advocacy
- Disease and health event investigation
- Screening
- Referral and follow-up
- Case management

Suggested Readings:
- **Edelman and Kudzma's** *Health Promotion Throughout the Life Span*
  - Chapter 4: The Therapeutic Relationship
  - Chapter 22: Young Adult
  - Chapter 23: Middle-Aged Adult
- **Nies and McEwen's** *Community/Public Health Nursing*
  - Chapter 31: Occupational Health
- **Stanhope and Lancaster's** *Foundations for Population Health in Community/Public Health Nursing*
  - Chapter 32: The Nurse in Occupational Health
- **Stanhope and Lancaster's** *Public Health Nursing*
  - Chapter 43: The Nurse in Occupational Health

Case Study Objectives:
After completing this case study, the student should be able to:
1. Describe the role of the occupational health nurse.
2. Discuss employment/health interactions and give examples of work-related illnesses and injuries.
3. Complete an occupational health history.
4. Discuss the federal regulations that apply to occupational health.

CASE STUDY 51

School Nursing

Case Study Synopsis: Nurse Peggy is a school nurse at XYZ high school. In a span of 2 years, she interviews for the job, provides direct care, performs outreach, develops school policy, and works on a coalition for school nurse legislation.

Estimated Completion Time:
- Case study only: 1 hour
- Plus review questions: + 30 minutes
- Plus discussion questions: + 15 minutes
- Total: 1 hour 45 minutes

Concepts Covered:
- Stress
- Coping
- Anxiety

Public Health Nursing Interventions Addressed:
- Outreach
- Health teaching
- Advocacy
- Policy development and enforcement
- Consultation
- Coalition building

Suggested Readings:
- **Nies and McEwen's** *Community/Public Health Nursing*
  - Chapter 30: School Health
- **Stanhope and Lancaster's** *Foundations for Population Health in Community/Public Health Nursing*
  - Chapter 31: The Nurse in the Schools
- **Stanhope and Lancaster's** *Public Health Nursing*
  - Chapter 42: The Nurse in the Schools

Case Study Objectives:

After completing this case study, the student should be able to:

1. Differentiate community health nursing and public health nursing within school nursing.
2. Explore the Framework for 21st Century School Nurse Practice.
3. Apply the roles of the school nurse to the care of children in the school setting.
4. Categorize care a school nurse provides within each level of prevention.
5. Explore the Coordinated School Health Program in the context of school health issues.
6. Incorporate integrative nursing principles to the care a school nurse provides.